Lithium and Lithium Carbonate

A medicinal product for Depression, Alzheimer and Dementia, for improving well-being and managing stress

Published by Expertengruppe Verlag

The contents of this book have been written with great care. However, we cannot guarantee the accuracy, comprehensiveness and topicality of the subject matter. The contents of the book represent the personal experiences and opinions of the author. No legal responsibility or liability will be accepted for damages caused by counter-productive practices or errors of the reader. There is also no guarantee of success. The author, therefore, does not accept responsibility for lack of success, using the methods described in this book.

All information contained herein is purely for information purposes. It does not represent a recommendation or application of the methods mentioned within. This book does not purport to be complete, nor can the topicality and accuracy of the book be guaranteed. This book in no way replaces the competent recommendations of, or care given by a doctor. The author and publisher do not take responsibility for inconvenience or damages caused by use of the information contained herein.

Lithium and Lithium Carbonate

A medicinal product for Depression, Alzheimer and Dementia, for improving well-being and managing stress

Published by Expertengruppe

TABLE OF CONTENTS

About the author

Lutz Schneider lives with his wife, Doris, in an old farmhouse in beautiful Rhineland.

Ever since he studied the biology of evolution, over 20 years ago, he has been interested in marginal health subjects, which are often hidden from the main stream, but which are scientifically well accepted. He teaches this knowledge, not only to his students, but also reaches a wider audience in Germany with his various publications.

In his books, he speaks about subjects, the positive effects of which are widely unknown and on which he can pass on his own experiences. All of his publications, therefore, are based on indisputable scientific facts, but also encompass his own very personal experiences and knowledge. This way, the reader not only receives factual information about the subject but also a practical guide with a wide range of knowledge and useful tips, which are easy to understand and put into practice.

Lutz Schneider's easy to read work puts the reader into a relaxed and pleasant ambience, while gaining insight into a subject which few know anything about but which everyone could profit from.

Preface

Lithium is mostly known for its use in batteries. Most people do not realise that it is also a trace element in our bodies. You can find it in small quantities in the Lymph nodes, organs and the brain. We also have some in our teeth, in combination with Phosphorus. We regularly consume Lithium in our food. You can find it mainly in whole grain foods and vegetables, such as onions, garlic and potatoes. There is also a small amount of it to be found in animal foodstuffs, such as eggs, butter and meat. If you follow a balanced diet, you will normally consume a certain amount of Lithium.

„Lithium makes us happy and healthy“[1]

---

[1]https://www.ddbnews.org/ddbnews-gesundheit/lithium-macht-uns-gluecklich-und-gesund/

I discovered this slogan during my early research for this book. It continues “Even small amounts of Lithium can reduce the risk of mental illness, such as Alzheimer and improve mood1. Similar to batteries, Lithium seems to recharge us too. To me, it sounded much like a magic potion but I remained sceptical and researched further into it.

In the following chapters I will explain in detail the results of my research. It will show that Lithium is an important component for all of us in achieving a lasting, healthy way of life. Clinical studies and scientific articles are speaking a clear language. Despite that, Lithium is suffering a niche existence by a large majority of pharmaceutical scientists and is hardly known by the broad population.

Even so, the advantages of Lithium, which lie in the psychological and mental health sector, are obvious and it is easy to obtain and use. I have taken care to maintain an abundant supply of Lithium in my body and have never experienced health problems. Lithium is not only essential for healing certain sicknesses, but also as a preventative element in everyone's diet.

What is Lithium and where does it come from?

Lithium is a chemical element with the symbol LI and the atomic number 3. It belongs to the group of alkaline metals and can be found in the second period of the periodic system of elements. It is a light metal and has the lowest density of all the solid elements. It was discovered in rock by Johan August Arfwedson in 1817 and this is how it got its name: Lithos means stone in Greek.

You can find Lithium in sea water and in the earth. This metal is used for many things in industry, for example in rubber manufacturing and the production of batteries.

Small amounts of Lithium are present in the human organism and Lithium salt is often found as a trace element in mineral water. However, this element is not vital and has no biological function, although it is proved to have a number of therapeutic effects, particularly from a psychological point of view.

Even back in ancient times, when depression was known as “cyclical insanity”, the sickness was treated in mineral springs rich in Lithium. This knowledge was lost in the middle ages. In 1850, Lithium was used as a treatment for gout and infections, but was found to be ineffective. After that, Lithium disappeared once again from the medical palette. From 1929 to 1950 the carbonated drink “7 Up” was enriched with Lithium and was touted as a mood enhancer.

It was not until 1949 that Australian psychiatrist, John F. Cade discovered, in a study, the anti-manic properties of Lithium salt. After he had injected guinea pigs with Lithium salt they reacted less strongly to external stimuli and were calmer, but not sleepy. After Cade had done some experiments on himself, the study of Lithium Carbonate was initiated for use as a medicine for the treatment of depressive, schizophrenic and manic patients, thus laying the foundation stone for Lithium therapy.

At the beginning of the 1950s, a Danish psychiatrist called Mogens Schou learned about the work of the Australian psychiatrist, John Cade. In further studies, he determined that Lithium could combat acute manic symptoms. Even more importantly, in a long-term study during the 1960s, Schou discovered that Lithium treatment could drastically reduce the number of manic and depressive phases. Since then, many studies have taken place to research the long-term and side-effects of Lithium.

What are Lithium salts?

In medicine, Lithium, in the form of Lithium salts is made into tablets. These salts are created by a chemical bonding/reaction with other elements. These salts include:

- Lithium Carbonate: This is a bonding between Lithium and Carbon. It is rarely found in nature and is therefore made from Lithium-containing ore and brines.

- Lithium Acetate: This is the Lithium in acetic acid. It can be made from a reaction with Lithium Carbonate or Lithium Hydroxide. Lithium Hydroxide in its purest form is normally only used in the production of lubricating grease.

- Lithium Citrate: This can be made from a reaction of Citric Acid with Lithium Carbonate.

- Lithium Sulphate: This is created by a reaction between Lithium Carbonate and Sulphuric Acid.

- Lithium Orotate: This is the Lithium salt of Orotic Acid, which is a chemical intermediate product which occurs during the production of DNA chains inside the cells.

The main supplier of Lithium is our nutrition. For example, 0.5 mg Lithium each is to be found in:

- 300 g eggs
- 500 g butter
- 500 g cereals
- 500 g rice

- 500 g meat
- 700 g milk
- 1200 g chocolate

In Germany, the average amount of Lithium absorbed per person is approximately 0.8 mg per day, and within the spectrum of 0 and 3 mg. The amount of Lithium we actually need is neither determined nor can it be accurately estimated. In a technical paper from 1960 it was estimated at 10 mg per day. It is not known if adverse reactions have occurred by a dosage of more than 10 mg Lithium.

Lithium is used in today's medicine to prevent repeated phases of depression and mania and to help in acute situations. It is also used for schizophrenia and cluster headaches. I will explain these medical conditions later in the book.

How does Lithium Work?

Lithium is a neuroleptic and anti-depressive drug. It effects countless processes in the human body at the same time. This is why its effect is largely unknown. For example, it has not been investigated as to why Lithium inhibits euphoria on the one hand, but on the other hand can brighten moods during depressions.

It is presumed that Lithium reduces the probability of further recurrences of affective episodes by reducing the noradrenalin excess during manic episodes and activating the production of Serotonin during depressive episodes.

It is also known that Lithium is enriched mainly in the white brain matter. There is an assumption that Lithium, in contrast to psychopharma-ceuticals, does not affect the transmission of signals to the synapses of the nerve cells, but in the nerve pathways themselves.

Lithium apparently also increases the release of both the GABA and Serotonin neurotransmitters.

GABA means Gamma-Aminobutyric acid or y-amino acid. These amino acids positively affect the human sense of wellbeing and performance. The most important job of the GABA is to pacify the neurotransmitters. It filters out the stimuli which cause stress in the body. The role of the GABA is to "relax the thoughts" contributing to a sense of inner tranquillity.

In addition, Lithium increases the Serotonin level in the body. Serotonin is a neurotransmitter and a messenger substance. It controls many processes in the human body, such as emotions, sense of pain and moods. This is why it is known as the "happiness hormone".

As described above, Lithium supports the release of these two substances which, in turn, makes us feel happier and more relaxed. However, it is not absolutely clear how this effect is reached.

In addition, Lithium helps in the de-activation of the ion channels, it blocks the cellular Natrium-Potassium current. It is thought that this reduces the central excitability of the brain. Furthermore, Lithium intervenes in the secondary messenger systems. It influences a series of enzymes, causing a reduction in specific enzyme products and their secondary products. There is also a reduction in the potassium concentration of the cells. This is important because people who suffer from manic-depressive illnesses show high concentration of potassium.

It is very unusual for an active substance to be released as a medication without knowing how it works. Physicians usually want to know how and under which circumstances an active substance works in order to protect themselves from unexpected surprises. The regulatory authorities have made an exception in this instance.

As you can see from the above, Lithium is, in many ways, a valuable helper in your body and mind. This is not only true for sicknesses but also in everyday life. Everyone can profit from an optimal Lithium level in their body in almost any situation. Unfortunately, most people in Germany do not consume enough Lithium through their diets to profit from these advantages.

Which sicknesses does lithium help with?

Lithium is a substance which takes care of our brains and which functions as a switch and warning system in the body. It is, therefore, very important that this organ works faultlessly. Lithium can significantly reduce our risk of psychological sicknesses, such as depression or schizophrenia.

In various trials, it could be proven that Lithium affects the brain cells. It can influence our mood positively and reduce the protein deposits which are responsible for the Alzheimer sickness. There has also been some success with Lithium in treating cluster headaches. Lithium also supports the body in creating the myelin sheath which protects the axons (the projection of a nerve which transmits electrical nerve impulses away from the cell body), similar to the insulation of an electric wire. As with electrical wires, it is possible that signals can be transmitted at breakneck speed. If the Myelin sheath (the protective layer) is damaged, this can lead to failure symptoms. Damage to this sheath plays an important role in diseases, such as multiple sclerosis or Parkinson.

Lithium is also said to facilitate the growth of "grey matter", which is responsible for intelligence, perception processes and motor abilities in humans. In addition, Lithium supports the so-called autophagy which are responsible for constant cell renewal. Lithium is said to have an anti-inflammatory effect and helps where insulin resistance is present.

At present, Lithium is mostly used in the treatment of bipolar disorders. Lithium compounds are administered during active phases to reduce the depressions. Predominantly, it is used to prevent a new illness phase after a depression and as a phase prophylaxis. Treatment with Lithium salts is much more effective than conventional pharmaceutical products, which are usually prescribed. In addition, the suicide rate sinks significantly while using Lithium compounds.

Lithium is also used during the active phases of cluster headaches and in-between attacks. Similar to its use with depressions, it is used to prevent further occurrences and to reduce pain during active phases.

Lithium can also be used in the early stages of Alzheimer or dementia in order to reduce the protein deposits in the brain. Unfortunately, no success has been recorded in advanced cases. Up to now, its use has not received much attention.

In morbus Parkinson and multiple sclerosis, Lithium has not been used much, even though, as described above, it supports the myelin sheath which could slow down the progression of the disease. It is presently available for use as an "add on" product in tried and tested therapies.

Below I will explain the briefly mentioned sicknesses in more detail.

Depression, Mania and Burnout

DEPRESSION

There are many forms of depression. Therefore, it is useful to recognise the various forms of such disorders and to know their symptoms. These adversely effect all aspects of life, including work and social relationships and can be light, moderate or severe. I would like to show you briefly, several different types of depression.

- Major Depression: Loss of interest and pleasure in normal activities and despondency are symptoms of major depression. These symptoms usually last at least two weeks and appear on most days. Major depression is a unipolar disorder as only the depressive phases occur.

- Psychotic Depression: People with depression sometimes lose their awareness of reality and suffer from a psychosis. This means that they suffer from hallucinations, delusions or believe that they are themselves evil and guilty of causing the negativity around them.

- Pre-natal and post-natal depression: During pregnancy (pre-natal period) and in the year after the birth (post-natal period), women are subject to an increased risk of depression. After the birth, there are hormonal changes which can cause the so-called "baby blues". Roughly 80% of women suffer from this. This condition, caused by the every-day stress of the pregnancy and caring for a new-born, is a normal experience. This is not the same as a clinical depression. A real depression affects not only the mother but also the baby, the partner and other family members. It also lasts longer.

- <u>Bi-polar disorder:</u> This type of depression is also called "manic depressive disorder" because the person affected suffers from depressive and also manic (excessive cheerfulness) phases. Between these phases, there may be a period of balance. In comparison to other mental illnesses, bi-polar disorder is often hereditary. Stress and conflicts can cause extreme mood changes. In addition, bi-polar disorder is often diagnosed wrongly. It is particularly difficult to diagnose if sufferers have not previously experienced any manic phases.

- Cyclothymic disorder: This is a less pronounced form of bi-polar disorder. Sufferers have chronic mood changes of a period of at least two years, where the symptoms of the manic phases and depressions are lighter to medium in strength. Between them there is a short phase of normality. The symptoms are shorter in length, less severe and not as regular.

- Dysthymia: This is a form of neurotic depression. It has the same symptoms as a major depression but is less pronounced, although it lasts much longer. A person is said to have

Dysthymia when he or she has this mild form of depression for more than two years.

- Autumn-Winter depression: This is a form of mood change which is linked to the seasons. It occurs mostly when Winter begins and stops when Winter ends. The disorder is usually diagnosed when the sufferer presents with the same symptoms for several years in a row. The symptoms include mood changes (depressive OR manic phases). Sufferers usually feel listless; they sleep and eat too much.

There are also many other kinds of depressions. It is often difficult to recognise one. There is a fluid line between normal gloominess and a light depression. Symptoms which indicate a depression are:

- Tendency to withdraw
- Restlessness
- Tiredness
- Insomnia, particularly in the second half of the night
- Lack of concentration
- Lack of interest in activities
- Lack of hygiene
- Inhibited libido
- Slower thought processes

If you suffer from one of these forms of depression, or if you recognise the symptoms mentioned above, Lithium is a possible way to achieve improvement.

MANIA

A mania is the opposite of a depression and can vary in strength. The sufferer always feels invincible, which is a reason why he or she does not want that condition to change. You can recognise mania by the following symptoms:

- You feel great or you are easily provoked
- You are full of energy and do not need much sleep
- You think extremely quickly, get floods of ideas and have delusions of grandeur
- You speak unusually quickly
- You behave erratically
- You have difficulty in concentrating.
- You are much more willing to take risks.

- You suffer from restlessness and nervousness.

In come cases the sufferer loses contact with reality. It can happen that the sufferer becomes a danger to him/herself or others. The sufferer could also develop an addiction to, for example betting.

Manic symptoms can also be significantly improved using Lithium.

BURNOUT

Burnout is not a depression but often a precursor to one. In the last few years, burnout has become a widespread disease, so I would like to refer to it briefly. The most common cause of burnout is stress. Hence the word burnout which is a synonym for exhaustion.

Burnout affects mostly those people you would least expect it to. They are in the prime of life, successful at work, have a family. Often, they are involved in club activities. They are active around the clock, goal-orientated. They are often managers or people with great responsibility at work.

The other target group for a burnout is more or less the opposite of that mentioned above. These are people with little confidence, are very emotional and sensitive and unable to withstand the pressures expected of them in today's world.

The symptoms of a burnout are similar to those of depression. There is a difference between physical and mental symptoms.

Physical symptoms:

- Sleeplessness and nightmares
- Tiredness and exhaustion
- Weight changes
- Weakening of the immune system
- Gastro-intestinal complaints
- Dizziness
- High blood pressure
- Pain in various parts of the body
- Loss of libido

Mental Symptoms:

- Increased irritability
- Impatience

- Helplessness
- Loss of memory
- Tendency to daydream
- Loss of concentration, even in small things
- Reduced resilience
- Tendency to withdraw
- Absence from work
- Lack of interest in activities

There are some other illnesses which have similar symptoms and must therefore be eliminated first. For example, hypothyroidism and senile hypothyroidism (under or over functioning of the thyroid glands). The consumption of various medicines, such as thyrostatic and anti-hypertonic substances or calcium blockers, can also produce symptoms similar to depression.

As you can see, in view of the wide array of sicknesses, it is difficult to make an exact diagnosis and therefore to clarify if Lithium alone is suitable to offer relief. A visit to the doctor or psychologist is often unavoidable. Don't be afraid to go. Helping yourself is the first step to a better life.

SCHIZOPHRENIA

Schizophrenia counts among the most serious of the mental illnesses as it influences the whole personality. Hallucinations, delusions, thought disorders and limitations in sensitivity are only a few of the symptoms.

Schizophrenia often comes in waves. The symptoms remain for a certain time and then, after weeks or months, start to subside. They can also disappear completely.

There are various forms of schizophrenia:

- Paranoid Schizophrenia is when sufferers believe they are being watched by aliens or ghosts and they talk to them. The often suffer from paranoia and hear voices, which give them orders. Paranoid schizophrenia is the most common form of schizophrenia and is characterised by constant and frequent delusions and hallucinations.

- Catatonic Schizophrenia presents mostly through movement disorders. Some patients become stiff or motionless. Others become very restless, for example rocking backwards and forwards with the upper body. Some obey all orders like a robot or do exactly the opposite to what they are told.

- A disorder which often shows itself in young people is a disturbance of moods and feelings. This is known as Hebephrenic Schizophrenia. The sufferer acts irrationally: cheerful, immature, silly, sometimes unpredictable or flippant. For example, he could laugh without reason. Often this is accompanied by thought disturbances.

- A very mild form of Schizophrenia is the Schizophrenia Simplex, which often develops insidiously. Concentration reduces, as does intellectual performance. Things which used to be important become less interesting. They tend to withdraw. Hallucinations and delusions do not occur in schizophrenia simplex suffers.

As mentioned previously, schizophrenic illnesses can also be treated with Lithium.

DEMENTIA AND ALZHEIMER

Alzheimer and dementia – are they not the same? No! Even when the cause of both is deterioration of the neurons and synapses, there are big differences between them.

Alzheimer:

Alzheimer is a cerebro-organic disease, which affects mainly people over 60 years old. The disease causes protein deposits (or plaques) in the brain. Typical symptoms are:

- Speech impediment
- Personality changes
- Memory loss
- Orientation disorders
- Impaired judgment

The symptoms increase with the advance of the disease and make normal life increasingly difficult until it becomes impossible.

<u>Frontotemporal Dementia (Pick's Disease)</u>

In contrast to Alzheimer disease, this form of dementia occurs normally between the ages of 50 and 60 years. It can also occur significantly earlier or later in life. The age range is between 20 and 85. With frontotemporal dementia the neurons and synapses in the forehead and temporal region begin to lessen. These control emotional and social behaviour. This means that the disease initially causes a breakdown in personality and interpersonal behaviour. As the disease progresses, it causes difficulties in finding words and understanding. This can lead to the sufferer becoming mute.

Alzheimer and frontotemporal dementia are the two most common forms of dementia. Added to that there are also:

- Creutzfeldt-Jakob Disease: caused by consumption of contaminated meat. This often presents in a combination with depression and leads to impaired movement, cognitive disorder and dementia.

- Vascular Dementia: This is described as old-age dementia and is similar in characteristic to Alzheimer.

- Korsakoff's syndrome: This starts like a dementia but is in fact an amnesia, often caused by poisoning, alcohol abuse or craniocerebral trauma.

As the various forms of Alzheimer and dementia have similar symptoms and causes, they can all be treated with Lithium.

CLUSTER HEADACHES

Untreated Cluster headaches are among the most severe and impeding pain diseases. They mostly appear as pain attacks with possible secondary symptoms, such as:

- Red and watery eyes
- Running or blocked nose
- Contracted pupils
- Hanging eyelids
- Sweating in the forehead area.

This disease mostly comes in waves. Individual attacks often come after falling asleep or in the early mornings.

MULTIPLE SCLEROSIS

Disseminated encephalomyelitis – also known as multiple sclerosis (MS) is a primary inflammatory disease which affects the central nervous system. The myelin sheath which covers the nerve fibres dissolves and is replaced by connective tissue. This leads to hardening and calcification.

The cause of this autoimmune disease (misdirected immune response – the body's own tissue is viewed as a foreign body) is not known to this day. MS presents in many different forms. Early symptoms may occur, such as impaired vision (seeing double), sensitivity disorders, an "electrifying" sensation when bending over, radiating throughout the body, slurred speech and trembling.

MORBUS PARKINSON

Morbus Parkinson, also known as shaking palsy, is when there is a reduction of dopamine-producing neurons in the brain. This leads to a dopamine deficiency syndrome. As with MS, the cause of Morbus Parkinson is not yet known in the majority of cases. It is assumed that the symptoms are caused by an imbalance between the messenger substance, Dopamine (also known as the happiness hormone) and Acetylcholine, which is responsible for transmitting stimulations of the nerves to the synapses in the central and peripheral nervous systems.

Trauma, brain tumours and inflammations of the brain are among the subordinate causes. The condition presents with rigor, tremors and akinesia. Rigor means stiffness/rigidity caused by increased muscle tone. Increased resistance when moving the extremities (cogwheel phenomenon) is a typical sign. Tremor means shaking, which is one of the first and most common symptoms. Excitement or agitation causes the tremor to increase. Akinesia means immobility. The patient has reduced ability or complete inability to move muscles in the face, torso or head. As the disease progresses, it can have serious consequences, including dementia.

It is not necessary to mention that the previously mentioned diseases of cluster headaches, multiple sclerosis and morbus Parkinson can also be treated with Lithium.

USING LITHIUM FOR ALS?

ALS (Amyotrophic Lateral Sclerosis) is a disease which affects the central and peripheral nervous system. The causes of this sickness are almost unknown up to now. One factor which could lead to this disease is possibly that it is hereditary. It is incurable and is a rare illness. ALS causes muscle weakness followed by muscular atrophy and usually death within 3 to 5 years. Often, however, people have survived for up to 10 years with ALS. The average age range for contracting the disease is between 50 and 70 years.

Perhaps you became aware of ALS through the so-called "ALS Ice Bucket Challenge" in the Summer of 2014, which flooded social media. Participants poured a bucket of ice water over their heads, after which they nominated further persons who had to repeat the action on themselves within 24 hours. If the nominee declined, he/she had to donate to the ALS Association (ALSA). Between 15th July and 27th August, 2014, the ALSA received 94.3 million US Dollars in donations, compared to about 3 million US dollars in the previous year. The ALSA recorded more than 2.1 million new donors.

But what does Lithium have to do with ALS? There are rumours that Lithium prolongs life in ALS patients. The reason for this is a study, made in 2008, where 44 ALS patients were given Lithium. The study was very promising, although there was no placebo group and the small number of 44 people who took the Lithium was not a representative study. After that, many universities carried out more representative studies, such as that of the Motor Neurone Disease Association of Great Britain and Northern Ireland. A total of 214 ALS patients took part in the study, but the results did not show a statistical significance in that case. The survival rate demonstrated very little change in life expectancy. There is presently no scientific evidence that the use of Lithium would extend life expectancy in patients with ALS.

Summary:

Medically proven!

Successful use of Lithium in acute medical conditions:

- *Depression and mania*
- *Dementia and Alzheimer*
- *Cluster headaches*
- *Multiple sclerosis*
- *Morbus Parkinson*

Why do you need Lithium?

Why do YOU need Lithium even if you do not suffer from any of the diseases mentioned above?

We are living in an ever faster-moving times. Stress is normal for most of us and it is easy to feel overwhelmed. It does not have to rise to the level of a burnout but we can still feel overstrained from time to time. Sometimes, a small trigger is enough: A difficult project at work, loss of employment often accompanied by financial problems, the death of someone close to you, a separation or even sometimes a small problem, such as a child's flu.

Lithium can also be applied in such cases, in order to help process stress situations. For such use, much less Lithium is needed as in, for example, a bipolar disorder and it can be obtained as a food supplement.

Lithium Orotate enables increased concentration and can also be used for chronic headaches, relief against epilepsy and as an aid during alcohol withdrawal. Positive effects were also observed in stimulating the immune system and as an antiviral agent (e.g. for herpes). However, since the 1980s, no meaningful research has been carried out with Lithium Orotate. In 2018, Dr. James Greenblatt, an expert in child and adult psychiatry, wrote: "...that side effects are non-existent when "lithium is used as a nutritional supplement." He continues: "Nutritional Lithium is a safe integrative strategy for the treatment of psychiatric and neurological disorders...and there are tremendous benefits related to many aspects of mood, behaviour and emotional health."[2] It makes us more contented and relaxed.

This also means that Lithium is not only successful in treating the disorders mentioned in the previous chapter, but can indeed also have a positive effect on the psychological and mental quality of every single person! It can even help in preventing the formation of these disorders.

Such consensually positive claims are seldom seen in other niches of medicine as they are with Lithium. To some extent it could be seen as a miracle cure. It is a natural substance which keeps our body and mind in a constantly balanced condition. It simply helps you to live happily and to protect you from sickness, such as depression and burnout.

---

[2] ZRT Laboratory Blog, dated 24th August 2017

How does Lithium help? What do you have to be careful of when taking it?

As already mentioned, Lithium is mostly used in the prevention and treatment of psychological disorders. According to recent studies, Lithium can also achieve good results when used for minor psychological disorders. It is possible to reduce aggressive behaviour by taking Lithium salts. Cluster headaches can also be effectively treated with Lithium salts.

It is interesting to note that, in May 2011, the "British Journal of Psychiatry" published a study from the Medical University of Vienna which showed that the suicide rate is lower where Lithium can be found in the drinking water. These values remain unchanged, even when taking into consideration other influencing factors, such as income or psychosocial aspects. The Austrian findings support the results of a study published in 2009 by a Japanese scientist.

In the German language article "Suizidprävention bei affectiven Störungen: Warum Lithium einzigartig erscheint" translated: "Suicide Prevention in affective disorders: Why Lithium seems so unique.", which was published in January 2019 in the magazine "InFo Neurologie & Psychiatrie", those effects appear to confirm previous findings. The article says that, taking into consideration 34 public and random studies of control trials versus Lithium, there was a 75% reduction in suicides (those resulting in death and unsuccessful suicide attempts) in the group of people who were treated with Lithium.

A study of the University of Jena, Germany, published in the "European Journal of Nutrition", confirmed that a higher content of Lithium in drinking water increases life expectancy. Dr. Michael Ristow examined the death rate in 18 Japanese communities. Water specimens were taken in each community and the Lithium content was tested. The trial confirmed that the death rate was considerably lower in those communities which had a high Lithium content in their water.

In the meantime, it has also been determined that psychological well-being can be influenced by Lithium. Intellectual performance can also be greatly increased while taking Lithium. In many cases it is not yet researched in detail how the positive effects occur, but the facts are indisputable.

Prescription Lithium

Before treatment with prescription Lithium can begin, several preliminary examinations are necessary. Above all, kidneys, thyroid glands and heart should be tested for stress and damage. As soon as the results arrive, the right compound should be chosen. There are many substances available alone on the German market which differ mostly in the dosage. There are also some restrictions to observe when choosing the correct medicine. Pregnancy, cardiovascular diseases or kidney problems must also be taken into consideration. Pregnant women should avoid Lithium treatment completely. Because Lithium is absorbed into breast milk, new born babies should not be stilled during treatment of the mother so that Lithium does not enter the blood circulation of the child.

Care should be taken to avoid interactions with other medications. Patience and perceptiveness are required while adjusting to the correct dosage. A great deal of sensitivity is necessary when treating disorders with Lithium. The perfect dosage is usually determined during the treatment. As soon as the treatment begins, Lithium levels in the blood should be tested regularly. These tests should be carried out weekly at the beginning of the treatment.

No significant loss of effectiveness has been reported through long-term use. Only discontinuing the treatment can lead to loss of effectiveness. In any case, this should not happen abruptly but treatment should be reduced slowly and evenly. This should always be carried out under medical supervision.

There is no danger of addiction when using medications based on Lithium, even after taking it for many years. A concentration of 1.2 mmol/l of Lithium in the blood should not be exceeded. Ideally, the blood value should be between 0.6 and 0.8 mmol/l. In general, the dosage will vary from person to person, which means that medical supervision is crucial. An overdose of prescription Lithium can quickly cause unwanted side effects, such as:

- Weight gain: This can be caused by increased fluid in the tissue, thyroid hypofunction and fat deposits. However, weight gain is primarily caused by an increase in appetite and lack of exercise. This counts for up to 10% of Lithium compound consumers.

- Gastrointestinal problems: Including nausea, abdominal pain, vomiting and diarrhoea.

- Increased Urination: The Lithium treatment can adversely impact the kidneys in their function of retaining urine which can cause them to excrete up to 8 litres of urine per day. This is very annoying, but at the same time it is important to replenish those fluids before the lack of fluids reaches a dangerous level in the body.

- Trembling: This is mostly a mild tremble but which can be very unpleasant, particularly in occupations where the hands are the subject of attention. The higher the Lithium dose, the stronger the tremble may be.

- Skin changes: Taking Lithium can cause itching or rashes. Drying out of the skin or temporary loss of hair are also possible.

There are many other possible side effects but these affect a very small proportion of patients (<1 %). The level of dosage also has a great influence on this. Even small amounts in excess of the patient's recommended dosage can lead to an overdose. The symptoms for this are:

- Decrease in concentration
- Slowing down
- Tiredness
- Weariness
- Thirst
- Urgency to urinate
- Abdominal pain
- Nausea, vomiting
- Diarrhoea

- Trembling
- Light sensitivity
- Muscle weakness and Muscle twitches
- Slurred speech

Should one or more of these symptoms occur, it is imperative to visit a doctor. Failure to do so could result in a Lithium poisoning. This presents as an intensification of the symptoms which, in turn, could lead to seizures or delirium. If Lithium poisoning is suspected, an emergency physician should be called immediately. This is one of the reasons why Lithium is only prescribed in very small doses and is not always the primary treatment for depression. Patients who overdose can cause themselves serious illness or even their own death. With patients who have suicidal tendencies, the use of Lithium should be carefully considered, even though it is said to have a suicide-inhibiting effect.

But before you start worrying about the above-mentioned side effects, be aware of the signals that your own body is sending. Then you can react to any adverse effects.

As is clear from the above, Lithium-based preparations are accompanied by many side effects. Of course, these may not occur and they show significantly fewer side effects than other psychotropic drugs. It is also the case that very small amounts of the preparation can show significant improvements in the condition which is being treated.

The low dosage reduces the side effects. As the use of this substance does not cause any problems to the majority of those using it, a therapy with Lithium salts can be recommended. Generally, the side effects appear quickly so that steps can be taken directly to avoid them. It is recommended to use Lithium compounds in the evenings so that you can sleep through the majority of the side effects.

Prescription Lithium is only used on adults because there are few empirical values available in long-term therapy with children and juveniles. Robert Findling carried out a study in 2015 on the effect of Lithium on children and juveniles between the ages of 7 and 17 years. 53 of the 81 test persons, who were all suffering from bipolar disorders, were given Lithium compounds. The other participants were given a placebo. After eight weeks a significant improvement was observed in those who had received the Lithium compound. This shows that also children and juveniles react positively to a Lithium therapy.

Prescription Lithium is only meant for the treatment of acute conditions. It is extremely high in dosage and can cause a broad spectrum of side effects. This is the reason that it is only available on prescription and that is a good thing. It is definitely unsuitable for preventative purposes or for optimising the body's natural Lithium level. Here I can only warn you to take it in consultation with your doctor.

There are many prescription-free Lithium compounds which are more than sufficient to optimise your own body's Lithium level in order to achieve the advantages described previously. It is important to differentiate between:

a) An acute condition (such as depression): Prescription Lithium with accompanying side effects.

b) Optimisation of your personal Lithium level, to improve psychological/mental health and performance and to increase general well-being: Prescription-free Lithium without side effects.

Prescription-free Lithium

As already explained, Lithium is administered in the form of Lithium salts. A study with Alzheimer patients showed that even a small dose of Lithium is enough for a therapy. The study with Alzheimer patients was carried out in the early stages of their disorder. For a period of one year, patients were given one dose per day (between 150 mg and 600 mg) of Lithium. After 12 months, a significant reduction of the protein deposits in the brain was recorded. During the period of the study, significant improvement in memory performance was also noticed.

The participants who were not given Lithium experienced loss of memory and an increase in protein deposits. In a comparison study, carried out over the same time period, patients were given 0.3 mg Lithium per day. The results, however, were very similar to those of the first study.

A similar study with Alzheimer patients in advanced stages of the condition unfortunately did not produce improvement in the participants.

It became clear that even small amounts of Lithium can produce significant improvement in the health of the participants. Lithium Orotate is also available prescription-free and is considered to be a food supplement. In 1973, Hans Nieper – a German doctor – discovered that Lithium Orotate only contains 3.83 mg of pure Lithium, whereas Lithium Carbonate contains 18.8 mg of Lithium per 100 g. The active ingredient in both substances is the same, but there is a significant difference in the dosage. Food supplements of Lithium Orotate usually contain 5 mg Lithium (for example from Lindens, Piping Rock or Swanson

Ultra). In comparison, QUILONUM, the first choice for treating bipolar disorders, contains 450 mg Lithium. The pure Lithium content is therefore about 90 times greater (!) than can be found in Lithium as a food supplement.

The recommended dose per tablet per day is about 5 mg. As explained in the above-mentioned study, this is enough to achieve the required result. The great advantage of having such a small dose is the fact that there are no (or very few) side effects. Similar amounts of Lithium are to be found in some mineral waters, such as Adelheid, Quelle, Bad Mergentheimer or Bad Liebenzeller Paracelsusquelle. If the dosage per day, as described above, is observed, normally no side effects will be noticed. Food poisoning will not occur as a result of using Lithium as a food supplement.

As long as there is no acute pre-existing illness, you should always use prescription-free Lithium. You will feel the difference just as quickly and the side effects are almost eliminated.

How do you know that you need Lithium?

As already described, Lithium helps with a number of illnesses, even though the reason for their effect is unknown. An increase in Lithium should be considered in people who are suffering from psychological disorders, alcoholism or mental instability. Also, people who suffer from gout or uric acid stones would benefit from an increase in Lithium.

A deficiency or increased requirement of Lithium does not always have to be the result of an illness. Sometimes, seemingly insignificant factors, such as continuing stress or sugar-free nutrition, can cause a deficiency in Lithium.

Why does this happen?

Our brain is always using Lithium. If it is exposed to constant or long-term stress, the requirement for Lithium increases dramatically. This could lead to a deficiency in Lithium. Our nutrition does not always fulfil the need for Lithium, in which case the requirement must be met in other ways.

How do you recognise Lithium deficiency?

The deficiency and its effects are largely unexplored. In animal tests, however, it could be determined that life expectancy, birth weight and fertility are reduced when a deficiency is present. Researchers also found that a number of psychological disorders can occur as a result of a Lithium deficiency, including aggressive behaviour.

You can see from these tests that, although an increase in Lithium can positively affect your body, a particularly low level of Lithium can also have significantly negative implications in your daily life.

As many people take too little Lithium by way of nutrition, you should think about doing something actively to increase your Lithium levels, not only because of its positive attributes on your body, but also to avoid negative effects.

There are sure to be more scientific discoveries made over the next few years which will back up these claims. This knowledge will most likely increase due to the spreading popularity of this substance.

Some Press Reviews on the Subject of Lithium:

"A preventative treatment with this simple and inexpensive substance has proved to be a blessing for many seriously ill patients!"

Mogens Schou

"We have repeatedly observed that Lithium is one of the few medications that can switch off suicidal thoughts in the long-term. There is no other medication which reduces suicidal thoughts and actions so distinctly"

Professor Michael Bauer, Direct of the Clinic and Polyclinic for Psychiatry and Psychotherapy in the Uniklinik Dresden

"Its ordinary nature is deceptive because it holds the power *to transform* lives"

James Greenblatt

Once again, a short summary:

Lithium is being used increasingly and for more illness. The results of the therapies speak for themselves, even if the way they work is not yet understood.

Outside of clinical therapies, however, Lithium also plays an important role in generating physical and mental balance and creating a feeling of well-being. This allows everyone to be able to work on themselves quickly and simply.

Instructions for Use

Lithium can not make itself. As already described, it is administered in the form of tablets of various dosages. It should be taken with water. Lithium cannot become addictive.

Prescription Lithium compounds, such as those based on Lithium Carbonate, may only be taken under medical supervision. Serious side effects may occur which cannot be underestimated. These could lead to anything between an overdose and a poisoning. Regular blood tests are unavoidable.

The situation is completely different with substances which are offered in the marketplace as food supplements. These contain a much lower dose of Lithium which will not cause any side effects. They can be bought online or in the Chemists. Most online products are imported from Great Britain. The selection of products online is small, the best known is from Lindens. Contrary to prescription Lithium, the food supplement should be taken in the morning in order to allow its effects to be felt during the day. As already mentioned, there are no problems with side effects.

Taking prescription-free Lithium is simple and does not need additional supervision as there are almost no side effects. Basically, it could be said: If you do not want to take it every day, then take it simply when you need it!

Homoeopathy: Lithium Chloratum

Lithium is administered as Lithium Chloratum in homoeopathy. However, this substance has little to do with the Lithium described in previous chapters. It is a companion salt to Schussler Salts and can be administered as ointments, globules and tablets. Lithium Chloratum works as a detoxifier – and so has a purifying function. Using it causes increase excretion of uric acid and urea.

For this reason, it is used for rheumatism and gout. Lithium Chloratum has also found application in the nervous and immune systems as well as thyroidal turnover. Lithium Chloratum has been particularly useful in treating afflictions of the small joints, such as hand, foot or knee joints, and also in the treatment of heart problems. Painful swelling and stiffening of the joints can also be treated, as can stabbing pains in the chest or palpitations. Inflammation and blockages in the kidney area, bladder and urinary tracts are further usages. In addition to all the above, Lithium Chloratum has a special connection to protein metabolism and is therefore recommended for use in the treatment of weak connective tissue, tissue hardening or thickening.

These typical disorders in the building up and re-building of the connective tissue are also to be found in Psoriasis. In chronic cases, Psoriasis presents a major challenge for the patient. Such patients develop depressive phases and psychological stress.

Lithium Chloratum does not only work on the protein metabolism but also within the nervous system. It supports mood swings, melancholy and psychological exhaustion. It has also proved helpful with stress-related eye and headaches. Lithium Chloratum enhances the absorption of Vitamin B12 and folic acid in healthy cells, it strengthens our immune system and has a restrictive influence on the growth of stubborn herpes and other viruses.

Lithium Chloratum can also be used in the treatment of inflammation of the mucous membrane, particularly by gastritis, and is also used to combat disorders of the digestive tract, such as flatulence and cramps. In the psychological field, it can be administered to counter fear of school or concentration problems.

As can clearly be seen, the scope of possible uses for Lithium Chloratum is very large. However, it does not have anything in common with the real Lithium therapy and cannot help in treating depressions, Alzheimer, cluster headaches or other such conditions. If you are suffering from one of the above conditions it is recommended that you visit the doctor. These conditions are not to be trifled with.

There are significant differences between the Lithium mentioned in the previous chapter and the Lithium Chloratum mentioned here. Do not allow yourself to be fooled! My explanations and the many positive uses of treatment strictly refer to the element Lithium!

Summary

The effectiveness of Lithium was only rediscovered during the 1950s. Despite that, it is being used to treat an increasing number of sicknesses. It helps with depressions, mania and Schizophrenia. It alleviates cluster headaches, can slow down the advance of Alzheimer and dementia and slows down the progress of multiple sclerosis and Parkinson. The results of the therapies speak for themselves, even when the reason for success is not fully understood. Lithium intervenes in many physical processes, whereby the side effects, such as weight gain, shaking and nausea are all possible. However, these side effects, and even worse ones, can also occur with other medications. Although the above-mentioned conditions cannot be healed with Lithium, they can be limited and even suspended. The consumption of these compounds should only be taken under medical supervision and regular blood tests are necessary during treatment.

This is not the case with prescription-free Lithium. This is mostly used to counter stress or emotional pressure. There are no side effects here.

Lithium has become an integral part of the treatment of depressive people, but much long-term research needs to be carried out in the areas of MS, Parkinson or dementia. Lithium as a food supplement can also be used to help with temporary stress, whether as a prophylactic or in acute stress situations.

Allow Lithium to become part of your everyday life – to become a habit. Then you can be sure that your body always has enough Lithium to keep your moods even and positive.

There is little discussion about Lithium but the medical evidence is unambiguous and shows that it is a significantly underestimated substance which could make our lives happier and more balanced.

Book Recommendations

LUTZ SCHNEIDER

THE POWER OF

BREATHING TECHNIQUES

Breathing Exercises for more Fitness, Health and Relaxation

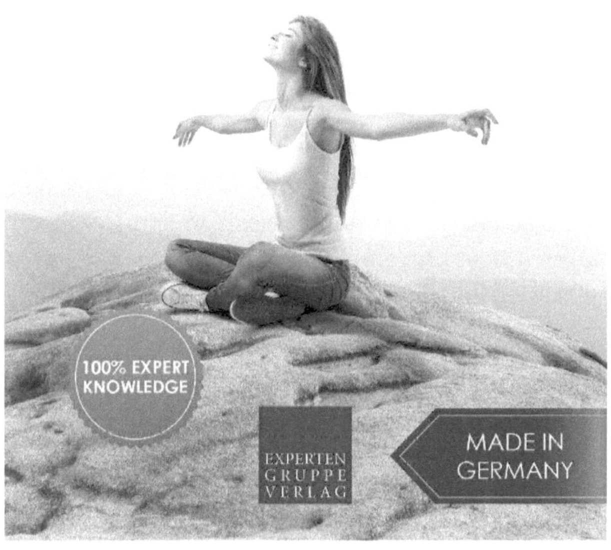

The Power of Breathing Techniques

Breathing Exercises for more Fitness, Health and Relaxation

We can survive for weeks without food and days without water, but only a few minutes without air.

Would it not be justified to presume that the air, which is more important for human survival than food or water, should live up to basic standards? How much air do we need for ideal breathing? And how should we breathe?

The amount of air that you breathe has the potential to change everything you believe about your body, your health and your performance.

In this book, you will discover the fundamental relationship between Oxygen and your body.

Increasing your Oxygen supply is not only healthy, it enables an increase in the intensity of your training and also reduces breathlessness. In short, you will notice an improvement in your health and more relaxation in your everyday life.

Look forward to reading a lot of background information, experience reports, step-by-step instructions and secret tips which are tailor-made to your breathing technique and help you to become fitter, healthier and more relaxed.

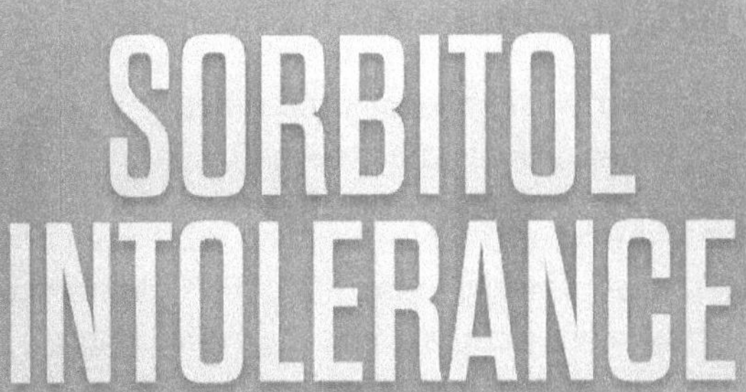

LIVING BETTER WITH SORBITOL INTOLERANCE – BACKGROUND, TUTORIALS, NUTRITIONAL ADJUSTMENT, RECIPES

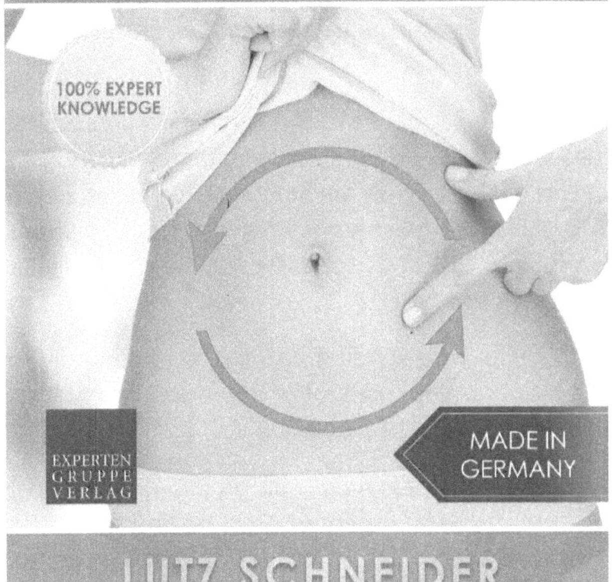

LUTZ SCHNEIDER

Sorbitol Intolerance

Living better with Sorbitol intolerance – background, tutorials, nutritional adjustment, recipes

Sorbitol intolerance is one of the least known food intolerances among many. And that, even though more and more people are suffering from it.

Wouldn't it be wonderful if you could at last find out if you suffer from Sorbitol intolerance? And how can you eat a diverse and delicious diet, despite your Sorbitol intolerance?

An increasing amount of industrially prepared food means that more and more people are taking doses of Sorbitol which they are not able to digest properly. This leads to a large number of lingering symptoms which are difficult to assign to any particular substance.

In this book you will find a simple guide on how to change your diet and a lot of important information about the subject of Sorbitol.

Read about fascinating background information, scientific findings, experience reports and secret tips which are tailor-made for you relating to your Sorbitol intolerance and which are designed to help you to achieve a healthy, longer and more fulfilling life.

Did you enjoy my book?

Now you have read my book, you know how best to live with your sorbito intolerance. This is why I am asking you now for a small favour. Customer reviews are an important part of every product offered by online shops. It is the first thing that customers look at and, more often than not, is the main reason whether or not they decide to buy the product. Considering the endless number of products available online, this factor is becoming increasingly important.

If you liked my book, I would be more than grateful if you could leave your review online.

Just write a short review as to whether you particularly liked my book or if there is something I can improve on. It will not take more than 2 minutes, honestly!

Be assured, I will read every review personally. It will help me a lot to improve my books and to tailor them to your wishes.

For this I say to you:

Thank you very much!

Yours

Lutz

List of references

Prof. Dr. med. Volker Faust: PSYCHIATRIE HEUTE: Seelische Störungen erkennen, verstehen, verhindern, behandeln.

Frank Herfurth, Bernhard Lenze: Ganzheitliche Ernährungsberatung: Ein Nachschlagewerk. Books on Demand 2014

Kim Zarse, Takeshi Terao, Jing Tian, Noboru Iwata, Nobuyoshi Ishii, Michael Ristow: European Journal of Nutrition: Low-dose lithium uptake promotes longevity in humans and metazoans. 2011

Konstantin Ingenkamp: Depression und Gesellschaft: Zur Erfindung einer Volkskrankheit. transcript Verlag 2014

James Greenblatt: Lithium - Das Supermineral für Gehirn und Seele: Effektive Hilfe bei:

Demenz, Parkinson, psychischen Störungen, Aggressivität, Ängsten, Sucht, ADHS. VAK Verlag, 2018

Maren Carbon: Suizidprävention bei affektiven Störungen: Warum Lithium einzigartig erscheint, erschienen in InFo Neurologie & Psychiatrie, Ausgabe 21. Springer Medizin 2019

Kerstin A. Gräfe: Bipolare Störung: Lithium auch bei Kindern wirksam und sicher, erschienen in Pharmazeutische Zeitung, Ausgabe 43/2015.

Marco Helbich, Michael Leitner, Nestor D. Kapusta: Lithium in drinking water and suicide mortality: Interplay with lithium prescriptions, erschienen in The British Journal of Psychiatry, Ausgabe 207. 2015

The ZRT Laboratory Blog
Lithium's Billion Year Journey: A Cinderella Story for Brain Health

Dr. James Greenblatt
August 24, 2017

https://www.welt.de/wissenschaft/article5028535/Was-Akkus-und-Depressionen-gemeinsam-haben.html

https://www.aerzteblatt.de/archiv/21213/50-Jahre-Lithiumsalze-in-der-Psychiatrie-Gibt-es-neue-und-bessere-Stimmungsstabilisatoren

http://www.drau-apotheke.at/?de/schuessler_salze/nr.16_lithium_chloratum

https://www.ddbnews.org/ddbnews-gesundheit/lithium-macht-uns-gluecklich-und-gesund/

https://www.deutsche-apotheker-zeitung.de/daz-az/2013/daz-31-2013/lithium-zur-behandlung-affektiver-stoerungen-und-als

All links have been opend lastly on February 08th 2019.

Disclaimer

1st Edition

 Publisher: GbR, Martin Seidel und Corinna Krupp, Bachstraße 37, 53498 Bad Breisig, Germany, email: info@expertengruppeverlag.de, Cover photo: www.depositphoto.com. The information provided within this book is for general information purposes only. It does not represent any recommendation or application of the methods mentioned within. The information in this book does not purport to imply or guarantee its completeness, accuracy, or topicality. This book in no way replaces the competent recommendations of, or care given by, a doctor. The author and publisher do not assume and hereby disclaims any liability for damages or disruption caused by the use of the information given herein

www.ingramcontent.com/pod-product-compliance
Lightning Source LLC
LaVergne TN
LVHW042259190726
843491LV00015BA/786

* 9 7 8 3 9 6 8 9 7 3 4 4 9 *